Pneumonia

A Simplified Handbook for Understanding, Preventing, and Managing Respiratory Health

Kelvin Braithwaithe

Table of Contents

Introduction

Welcome to a simplified, comprehensive guide designed to empower healthcare professionals and individuals alike to understand, prevent, and manage pneumonia. Pneumonia, an inflammatory condition affecting the lungs, remains a significant global health concern, demanding heightened awareness and informed strategies for prevention and treatment.

In this book, we discuss pneumonia, going over the pathophys, the different ways we can classify pneumonia based upon the microbes, how to acquire it, the location of some of the features and complications, and later about diagnostics and some treatment.

This handbook is valuable, offering a nuanced exploration of pneumonia's causes, symptoms, and risk factors. From the basics of respiratory anatomy to the latest advancements in medical research, this guide aims to bridge the gap between medical expertise and public knowledge. Whether an enthusiastic reader, a healthcare practitioner seeking up-to-date clinical insights, or an individual eager to safeguard respiratory health, this handbook provides information, practical tips, and evidence-based recommendations.

Join us on a journey through the intricacies of pneumonia as we unravel its complexities and equip the reader with the knowledge to make informed decisions. Together, let us navigate the path towards a healthier, pneumonia-resistant future.

Chapter One: Causes of Pneumonia

Let us start with the pathophysiology behind pneumonia. Whenever patients develop pneumonia, there are different mechanisms to develop it. Pneumonia is an inflammation infection of the lung tissue due to a particular pathogen. It could be bacterial, viral, fungal, or many different entities. The most common, though, is going to be bacterial.

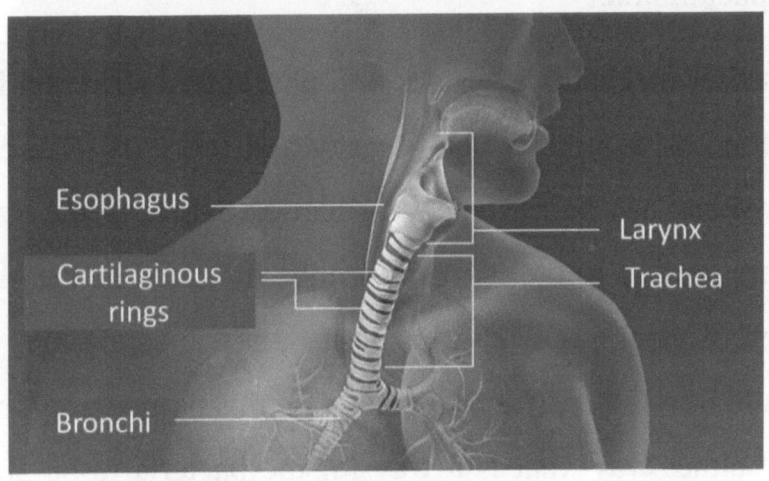

The ways that the bacteria get into the respiratory tract are important, and one of the ways that this can happen is usually aspiration. By aspiration, this usually means some type of secretion, whether this be like secretions within our oral pharynx and some of the salivary secretions and things from our oral cavity, nasal cavity, all of those things draining down, unfortunately, into the airway. So, oropharyngeal aspiration tends to be one of the most common ones. Some of the secretions within the oral pharyngeal portion, instead of going down into the esophagus, unfortunately, go right down into the airway. Furthermore, whenever these pathogens that are within these secretions get sucked up down into like a little bronchial or alveoli, they can cause damage to the lung tissue, inflammation of the lung tissue, infect it, and then lead to pneumonia.

Another mechanism besides oral pharyngeal secretion is the second aspiration, which is nasty and scary, is gastric. So, someone has some type of situation where some gastric secretions go right into their air tube. It would be the gastric type of aspiration. If someone has gastric aspiration, there could be a lot of different reasons for this particular problem, but either way, that is a way for the bacteria to be able to move from parts of the gastrointestinal (GI) tract, our esophagus, from our stomach, some of the natural flora within that area naturally to get into the lung tissue, cause injury, inflammation, infection, and then cause pneumonia.

Thus, the common question is, how would these particular pathogens from oral pharyngeal or gastric secretions even get into the lung tissue? How does it get into the airway? That is because we should naturally have protective reflexes to prevent that. Imagine trying to stab the back of the tonsils or the throat; it is going to have a gag reflex. Alternatively, something gets in the proximal airway, agitates the tissue there and creates some cough reflex. Instead of oral pharyngeal secretions or things coming from our GI tract going upwards into the airway that should naturally go down into the GI tract and follow the normal swallowing process, those should also all be intact. However, what if a patient does not have those intact?

Within our central nervous system are the parts that control many of these particular reflexes. Suppose many cranial nerves are involved in some gag reflexes, particularly within the cough or swallowing reflex. Moreover, if the patient has a disease process for whatever particular reason, some type of disease process or depression, whatever it may be, that is shutting down this cough gag and swallowing reflex. So, in these patients, the primary reason by which they aspirate is,

- the loss of the gag reflex or a decrease In the gag reflex,
- a decrease in the cough reflex or

- a decrease in the swallowing reflex.

That prevents us from being able to prevent things from going into the airway and also prevents us from naturally allowing things to go into the GI tract and then undesirably go right into the airway, creating an opportunity for pneumonia.

Thus, the question is, what kind of things would cause this disease process where it inhibits this? The simple answer is central nervous system (CNS) diseases. So, if a patient has any kind of CNS disease, for example, a stroke, damaged part of the brain, seizures, Parkinson's disease, ALS, multiple sclerosis—lots of different diseases are going to lead to the inhibition of the pathway from the brain., The other one is any kind of CNS depression, and this is important also to remember. So it may not be a disease process, but maybe the patients who are on some type of opioids or they are also taking particularly maybe some type of benzodiazepine, or they are being sedated, or they are being paralyzed because of the ventilator, or they have to be intubated, whatever; taking away the natural type of reflex from the central nervous system. So, any type of CNS depression would also be a big one. Another big one to remember is alcohol use as well. So alcohol use is a big one, as well as any kind of sedation. So remember that using sedation or neuromuscular blockade, things of that nature, either way, is shutting down the cough, gag, and swallowing reflex, allowing for aspirated material.

The bacteria involved

When these kinds of things happen, they let the microbes get in. What are some of the microbes that we should be concerned with whenever a patient aspirates? There are a lot of different bugs, but the ones, especially in patients with some type of underlying aspiration to be somewhat concerned with, and the microbes in this particular scenario—is Klebsiella. So, Klebsiella is a nasty bug. It is very common in patients who are in alcohol use or have some type of aspiration from a CNS disease. Other ones would be anaerobes. Why anaerobes? Because this will come from the GI tract. Naturally, the GI tract will have a lot of anaerobic bacteria. Furthermore, the other one to also consider is Staphylococcus aureus. So, the ones to potentially consider in patients who have some type of aspiration would be

- Klebsiella,

- anaerobic bacteria, and

- potentially Staphylococcus aureus

due to aspiration, loss of or decreasing gag, cough, or swallowing reflex due to CNS disease or CNS depression of some particular etiology.

What will be another reason a patient has a pathogen get into the airways, cause inflammation, infection, and lead to pneumonia? One way is to inhale a nasty kind of hardy pathogen, and what would that potential pathogen have to be? What would be some of the risk factors that would be associated with it? Suppose in a population, particularly in an environment with a high volume population, there is close contact with many highly populated individuals. There is the risk for some particular types of pathogens worth remembering, and the ones to potentially think about in situations where there is lots of close contact, many people hoarded together within a very tight population, is Mycoplasma pneumonia. It is a big one, Mycoplasma. Others include Chlamydia and potentially Influenza, and sometimes Legionella as well. So, these are things to consider in these particular patient populations. So, whenever in close contact, there is an opportunity for a lot of these particular pathogens to be passed on via respiratory droplets, inhaled, move right into the airway, and have the ability to cause a particular infection.

With Legionella, consider contaminated water sources, which could be in highly populated areas: hot tubs, pools, showers, air-conditioning units within many different hotels and things like that. So, there is aspiration and inhalation, particularly within close contact with airborne pathogens.

Possible fungal infections

There is another one: maybe it is not like a person-to-person transmission via Mycoplasma, Chlamydia, Influenza, or Legionella. Maybe it is some type of soil or dust exposure or nasty droppings from particular animals that put these patients at high risk, and it is dependent upon the geographic location, which is very high yield. It includes fungal infections, especially in the Southwestern portion of the United States, called coccidiomycosis.

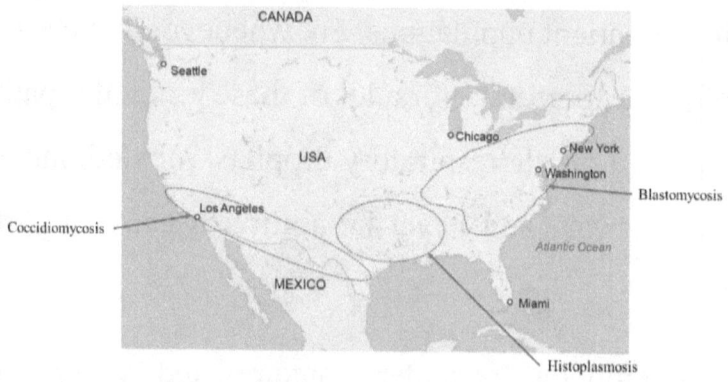

Whenever the patients say they were doing much spelunking, they were looking at different birds and bats and stuff like that near the Mississippi or Ohio River Valley areas, think about histoplasmosis. The next one is about broad-based yeast in the Eastern United States, which will be Blastomycosis. These are the particular fungal infections to be aware of and potentially airborne inhalation. So, these are the big things to be aware of for the potential etiologies: aspiration and inhalation.

Nevertheless, what if a patient, for whatever reason, does not have any particular problem with maybe an aspiration or an inhalation, but they have other kinds of problem that have to do with their normal respiratory function because they have underlying types of diseases that are altering their natural immune system defences, such as mucociliary clearance?

8

that potentially could be another problem for patients that are developing pneumonia.

Mucociliary clearance

If a patient does have no problem where they did not aspirate something, they did not have any situation where they inhaled like a hardy pathogen like a fungal infection or a Mycoplasma, Chlamydia, Legionella, or viruses, then is there something wrong with the actual anatomy of the respiratory tract? Is there a defence system that is slightly altered in a particular way? Thus, one of the big defence mechanisms that our respiratory tract has is mucociliary clearance, a really interesting concept.

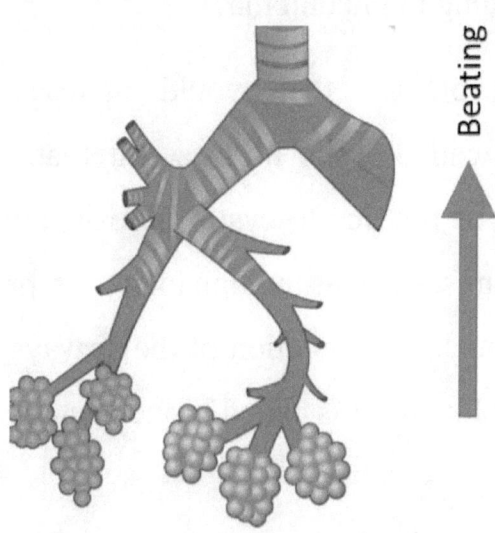

The cilia usually beat things upwards, so if something is stuck within the bronchi or the trachea, they will generally beat the bacteria and mucus upwards so we can spit it out or swallow it so it does not stay within the respiratory tract. Furthermore, sometimes, little mucus globules trap the pathogen again, making it easy to beat that bacteria via the cilia. Suppose there are disease processes that either chalk up the mucus where the cilia cannot handle all this mucus. Thus, they are trying to beat against the thick mucus wall, or there is damage to the cilia. Consequently, they cannot move that mucociliary clearance or escalator. What disease processes would alter this and lead to an opportunity for pathogens to get locked up in the lower airways, causing inflammation and infection, leading to pneumonia?

One disease process that would increase this mucus production is called cystic fibrosis. Alternatively, there are diseases, maybe not due to cystic fibrosis, but due to other particular things such as malignancies or primary ciliary dyskinesia, much inflammation of the airways, which could be something like what is called bronchiectasis.

In these particular situations, this will increase the mucus a lot. If there is an increase in the mucus, the cilia will not be able to beat the bacteria and all that mucus upward because the mucus will get so thick.

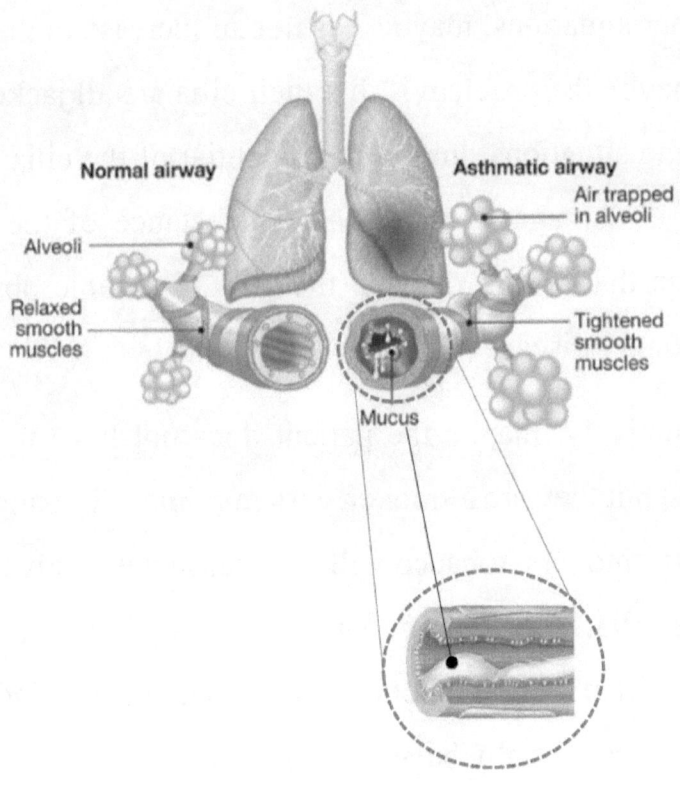

Imagine that these cilia are trying to be able to push like 2,000 pounds versus like 10,000 pounds; they have this big thing that they have got to try to move that is not going to allow the bacteria to be easily cleared. Plus, it will create an opportunity for bacteria not to get moved. So then what happens is some of these nasty little pathogens that are supposed to get cleared just stay in those areas, and then they move down to the smaller bronchioles and alveoli and create an infection.

In other situations, maybe it is not an increase in the mucus, but maybe the problem is that their cilia are all jacked up or, in some situations, inhibit the potential of the cilia. What if there is damage to the cilia? An instance of the kind of disease that would damage the cilia is chronic obstructive pulmonary disease (COPD).

Alternatively, maybe the patient does not have underlying COPD but they are a smoker. So sometimes, for patients who are big smokers, tobacco will also cause destructive damage to the cilia. Furthermore, as we age, aged individuals lose some of that natural function of the cilia. So, aged individuals will also potentially have this high risk.

Thus, what kind of microbes would be present if the cilia are not beating or the mucus is getting too thick? It creates an opportunity for the bacteria not to get mobilized. They stick down, and they cause pus to form, and then they lead to infection and pneumonia. There is potential to be aware of the potential within that situation.

- It is vital to be cautious, especially with COPD patients. So, patients who have COPD are at a very high risk for Hemophilus influenza and Moraxella catarrhalis. These are nasty types of bugs that can accumulate and cause infection.

- The others are patients who are going to have cystic fibrosis and bronchiectasis. These are at a high risk for a nasty bug called Pseudomonas aeruginosa. Smokers and aged individuals are at very high risk for another type of pathogen, particularly Legionella. Remember, it may also have to deal with the contaminated water sources. Nevertheless, this is also an atypical pathogen in patients who are smokers and aged.

These are situations where there is a problem where the patient aspirates. They aspirated some of these particular pathogens into the airway because of the alteration in their natural central nervous system function, inhaling a nasty pathogen because of close contact, or being in a particular geographic location that put them at high risk for a fungus.

They have some type of alteration within the normal defence system of the respiratory tract, like impaired mucociliary clearance.

Pneumonia in the bloodstream

What if, in some terrible situation, a pathogen gets into the bloodstream? When it gets into the bloodstream, it then spreads to the lungs. That would be a terrible situation. Patients who are IV drug abusers are very high risk, and whenever they are using dirty needles, for instance, on the skin, they have a potential pathogen called Staphylococcus aureus.

So, patients who are IV drug abusers have this risk of taking this pathogen from dirty needles, getting it into the bloodstream, and spreading it to the lung tissue, where it can then cause inflammation and infection. It can also lead to endocarditis and other problems, so consider Staphylococcus aureus in patients who are IV drug abusers.

The other thing to think about with Staphylococcus aureus is not just from IV drug abuse, but sometimes, in a patient population where they just had influenza. After they have influenza, their immune system is less protective, and they are at high risk for Staphylococcus aureus. So, post-influenza infections, these patients are at high risk for Staphylococcus. So, remember two things: IV drug abuse and post-influenza for Staphylococcus aureus. Thus, that is another way that patients can develop pneumonia. They can aspirate, inhale, or lose their mucociliary clearance, or it gets in the blood and spreads to the lungs.

What if the patient gets it spread from the blood? So, it comes from the blood, gets into the lungs, or is inhaled, aspirated, or impaired mucociliary clearance, and it gets in. Either way, the result is the same: the patient develops inflammation, infection, and pneumonia.

Immunocompromised situations

Our natural immune system provides another defence. We have macrophages where our immune system will come and try to clear and get rid of the pathogen and get rid of all that kind of infected material, which is a natural kind of immune response. However, what if a patient does not have a good immune system? What if, for whatever reason, their macrophages are not doing very well when they become exposed to that actual pathogen? They try to recruit a lot of lymphocytes and neutrophils, but all of this is particularly depressing. So, their ability to work and clear this infection, all of these immune system cells, is inhibited because their immune system is depressed. They have a decreased function of their macrophages, particularly a decreased number of lymphocytes, which would be the big one.

Furthermore, it just decreases the activity of the immune system in general. The kind of patients with this sort of particularly immunocompromised system include those with HIV and diabetes, maybe they have chronic kidney disease (CKD), alcoholics, and maybe they are status post-transplant. Alternatively, maybe they are on some type of immunosuppressant medication. Some types to be aware of include tumor necrosis factor (TNF) -alpha inhibitors, disease-modifying antirheumatic drugs (DMARDs), and any actual types of steroids.

Microbes that patients are at really high risk of when they are immunocompromised are also really important. So, if a patient is immunocompromised, they are at high risk for many different microbes, especially Pseudomonas.

Pseudomonas is very high risk in these patients with underlying disease processes and immunosuppression.

Another one, especially in this patient population, is Legionella. It is an atypical pathogen with contaminated water sources, aged, and smokers. Another one is the Pneumocystis jirovecii (PJP). It is a fungus, and the big population is patients with HIV(CD4 count less than 200). It is a PJP that's causing the pneumonia. So, a patient who is immunosuppressed with HIV, with a CD4 count less than 200, is exposed to this pathogen. Some viruses like Cytomegalovirus (CMV) and other nasty fungal infections sometimes exist. So, the major ones are Pseudomonas, Legionella, PJP, CMV, and potentially other fungal infections.

So, a good understanding of how patients can develop pneumonia includes,

- It could be from an aspiration problem,
- it could be from an inhalation problem,
- it could be from an impaired mucous clearance problem,

- it could be because it spread via the blood to get to the lung tissue, for example, with drug abusers or

- it could be because they got it from the blood or inhaled, aspirated, impaired mucous area clearance, or any of these mechanisms. However, their immune system was not competent enough to clear the infection.

Acquired pneumonia

When discussing pneumonia, it concerns pathophysiology mechanisms and microbes, but usually not about acquiring pneumonia. However, there are also instances of community-acquired pneumonia and hospital-acquired pneumonia.

- Community-acquired pneumonia (CAP): the pathogen emanates from the community, which means it is a special type of bug, for example, Streptococcus pneumonia. So whenever a patient has Usually, it is common with aged patients as well. They are usually acquired within the community, or they got admitted into the hospital, and within less than two days in the Hospital (Note: it has to be less than two days in the hospital) or out in the community

18

- If it is hospital-acquired, there is usually a very specific definition. Hospital-acquired pneumonia (HAP) has been in the hospital for more than 48 hours (more than two days), and the bug has changed from strep-pneumo to very resistant bugs encountered in the hospital. Moreover, usually, the most common type of HAP is a subtype called ventilator-associated pneumonia (VAP). These patients have an endotracheal tube or some type of trach within their airway. Once they are in the hospital for over two days, they will have nasty bugs they can form. And the two bugs to remember are,
    1. methicillin-resistant Staphylococcus aureus (MRSA) and
    2. the other one is Pseudomonas.

Now, in patients who develop ventilator-associated pneumonia because they have an endotracheal tube, they need that in more than two days to have the actual diagnosis.

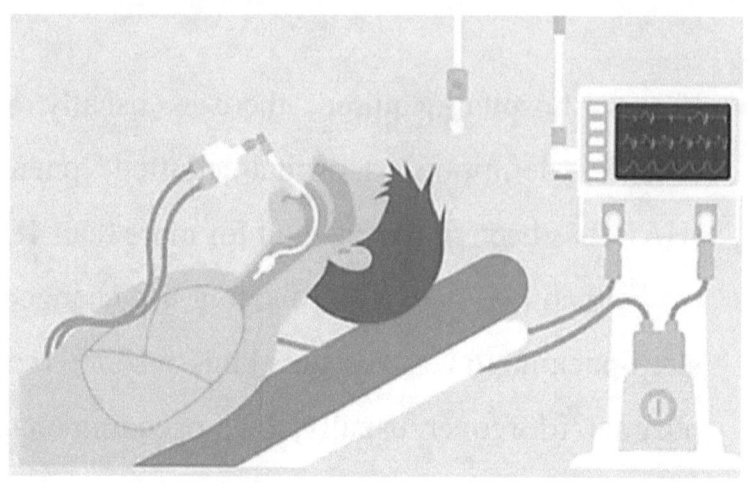

One huge consideration will be the potential things that put these patients at risk because of its relatively high yield. Often, when patients are in the ICU, we give them particular drugs to suppress their gastric acid production to prevent them from getting stress ulcers. We may give them things like proton pump inhibitors and Histamine H2 Receptor antagonists (H_2RAs) like famotidine. Moreover, that suppresses their gastric acid production so they do not get ulcers. It also increases the gastric pH, and bacteria survive better at a high pH. If that is the case, and for whatever reason, they reflux some of this around the edges of the endotracheal tube, and it gets into the lungs, which can cause a little nasty pneumonia. So, remember that gastric acid suppression is a big potential cause for ventilator-associated pneumonia.

Another case is when patients are being sedated. Normally, the patient can cough and clear those secretions or get suctioned if pathogens exist. However, if patients are not getting actively suctioned, there is decreased suctioning of potential secretions that can build up, form a film, and lead to an infection. Also, when patients are on lots of sedation, they do not have enough cough reflexes to clear many of those secretions. Another condition is if they are paralyzed and cannot cough. Thus, whenever they are not getting the secretions suctioned out or getting them to cough or taking away their cough and their natural mechanisms to clear secretions, such as increased sedation or increased paralysis for whatever reason, these potential things increase the risk of ventilator-associated pneumonia. However, they need an endotracheal tube for two days, then they think about these particular bugs for CAP.

Chapter Two: Features and Complications

When a patient develops pneumonia, they have an infection of their lung tissue. Whenever they start having this infection of their lung tissue, it is important to understand those features and complications that point towards pneumonia. There is typical pneumonia, which most people think is like a very specific bacteria subset, for example, Streptococcus pneumonia, Klebsiella, Hemophilus influenza, Staph aureus, Pseudomonas and others.

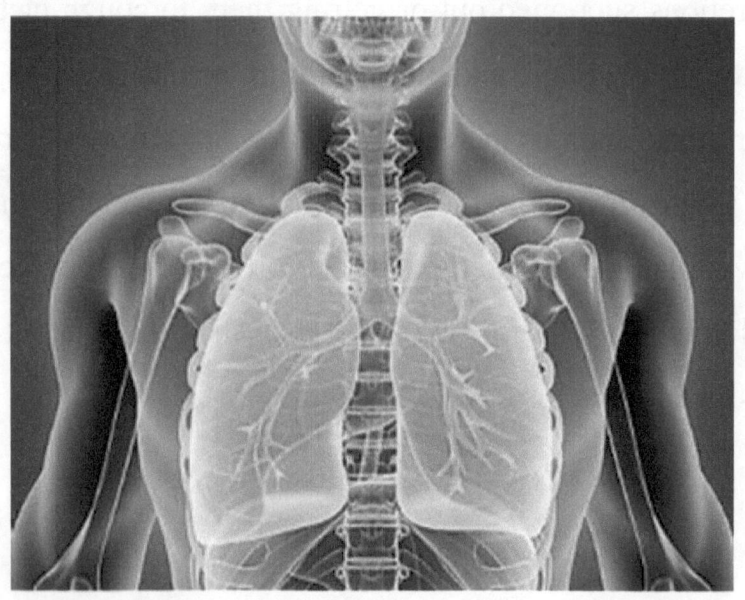

Atypical pneumonia

So, when discussing atypical pneumonia, it is about a very specific subset. Atypical pneumonia refers to a specific subset: Mycoplasma, chlamydophilia, and Legionella (MCL); these are the three atypical pathogens to remember.

The other ones to remember are viruses: influenza, parainfluenza, CMV, SARS-CoV-2, and COVID-19. So, there are a lot of different viruses out there that could also fit within the atypical umbrella. The key thing to remember is that with atypical pneumonia, due to Mycoplasma, chlamydia, Legionella, or viruses, they will not present with many of the classic features of typical pneumonia. The key way to differentiate this subset is that they present with upper respiratory tract infection-like symptoms. So, the atypical types of pneumonia due to these pathogens present upper respiratory tract infection-type symptoms. These symptoms include

- headaches,
- some type of nasal congestion or rhinorrhea,
- some type of sore throat,
- ear aches.

So, especially with mycoplasma pneumonia, it can cause a nasty tympanic membrane infection and cause bullous meningitis.

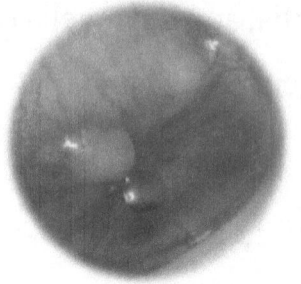
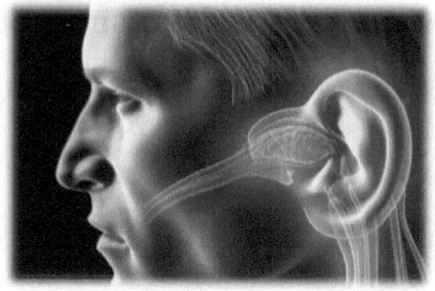

Upper respiratory tract infections may sometimes have very low-grade fevers, myalgias, and arthralgias.

Typical pneumonia

For the typical pneumonia it shows a lot of classic features. Whenever a patient has an area of infection, so all of the lower part of the lung is locked up with bacteria, it will cause a massive inflammatory process which releases many cytokines- interleukin-1, interleukin-6, and more.

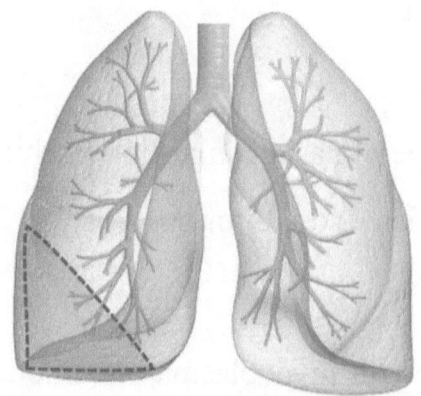

However, what they do is the central nervous system, particularly at the hypothalamus level. The hypothalamus tries to increase the body temperature so that the bacteria cannot survive, and so the patient may develop fever and rigors, very common features in patients with atypical pneumonia. Moreover, it would be important to remember that it would be more of a high-grade rather than a low-grade fever. The other thing is that it will lock up little alveoli with pus and even maybe hit some bronchioles.

Normally, when we have a good oxygenation measurement, it depends upon the alveoli's ventilation and the alveoli's perfusion. Suppose, in this situation, the perfusion is normal. So, the ability to move blood through the pulmonary vessels and pick up oxygen is good. However, the ventilation in this situation is decreased because sending oxygen into the locked-up alveoli is difficult because the oxygen has to try to move across these all socked-up and pus-filled alveoli. So, imagine how little oxygen is going to move into the alveoli. So, the result is low ventilation and normal perfusion, a combined effect called a V-Q mismatch. Moreover, whenever there is a V-Q mismatch, this can lead to hypoxemia due to the alveoli being filled with pus. When a patient gets hypoxemic, they show some of the potential reflexive reactions that may be present on the vital signs.

25

The patients coming in have high-grade fevers; they got rigors. They have low O2 saturation on their pulse ox. So, whenever there is a locked-up area, that causes that VQ mismatch. So, decreased ventilation to the portion of the lung whenever there is a mismatch in that portion due to decreased ventilation and good perfusion leads to hypoxemia, resulting in low levels of oxygen within the blood.

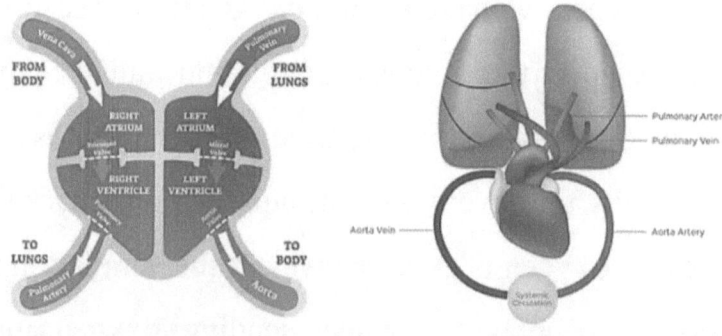

When that gets into the pulmonary circulation, it will go back to the left side of the heart because the pulmonary veins return to the left heart. Moreover, it empties all that blood into the left ventricle when it returns to the left heart. It will take this blood from the left ventricle and then send it outwards into the aorta and the Carotid system. All the chemoreceptors within the aorta and the Carotid bifurcation pick up the sensation of oxygen and the concentration of oxygen. Moreover, whenever the oxygen concentration is low, it activates these chemoreceptors, sending sense impulses into the central nervous system. When the medulla senses that the oxygen is low, it responds by increasing the blood flow from the heart to the lungs to increase perfusion and the need to increase the respiratory rate to increase ventilation. Thus, subsequently, the patient may have an increase in their heart rate, and they also may have an increase in their respiratory rate and depth. So, they may present with dyspneic and tachycardic hypoxemic fevers and rigors. Suppose some of the pneumonia involves some of the actual bronchi and bronchioles, and the patient has some pus filling the lungs and the alveoli. Whenever the bronchi and bronchioles get inflamed, they are heavily innervated by many noisy receptors, like cough receptors. Thus, they will go haywire when stimulated by much inflammation, sending that information into the central nervous system. In response, the central nervous system assumes there are a lot of secretions and mucus within the airways and may be able to clear some of those secretions up with coughing. Thus, it produces this intense cough reflex to ensure the cough is productive. So with these patients, look for a productive cough filled with a lot of mucopurulent sputum, high fevers, rigors, hypoxemia, reflexive tachycardia, and tachypnea, which may look like they are breathing hard and working hard to breathe.

Suppose there is inflammation of the lung parenchyma, which gets close to involving the nearby pleura; agitating or inflaming the pleura also triggers the Pain receptors near that pleura. These agitation receptors can pick up that sensation of inflammation and send that to the central nervous system. Moreover, these somatic motor fibres present with the referred type of pain. Thus, they will have pain in their chest whenever they take a breath, called Pleuritic chest pain; it is very common in any type of pulmonary pathology to present with pleuritic chest pain. So look for pleuritic chest pain, productive cough, hypoxemia, reflexive tachypnea, tachycardia, high-grade fevers, and rigors.

Suppose a patient gets a locked-up portion of the lung, say a big old consolidation in their lung. Maybe it is filled with fluid, that is filled with pus, that is filled with cells. All of those things are kind of fluid consolidation. Take, for instance, whenever sound moves through particular substances; if it moves between air and fluid, which one would it move faster and better? It moves better and faster through the fluid than it does the air, and so it increases the intensity of a lot of physical exam findings. So, one of the things that would be very, very important to consider is when percussing on the patient's chest, it produces the sound, something called dullness to percussion. So, there will be much dullness to their percussion. When examining a patient, listen with the stethoscope put over their chest and have them perform some specialized activities; the first thing is to have them say some word, for instance, '99,' and listen to their lungs or where the area of consolidation is. When that sound is moving through the consolidation when they say '99,' it will sound so dang clear, and it should not sound clear. So, because of the air that usually fills that space, if they have what is called 'able to hear the 99 clearly during auscultation', that is called positive bronchophony.

The other one is that sometimes, to have the patient say 'e,' and when they say 'e' or whenever the sound moves through that consolidation, it amplifies it and changes to where it can sound like 'a.' So, if it goes from 'e' to 'a, ' that is consistent with a consolidated finding. So, we call that positive egophony. Remember, 'e' goes to 'a,'. Another test is to have

29

them whisper, and so when only having them whisper things like, 'one, two, three.' what that will do is that it should not be audible at all in a patient who has all air-filled lungs.

Nevertheless, if they have a consolidation, that sound will move easily and relatively audibly. So, if it is audible to hear 'one, two, three' when they whisper easily, it is consistent with consolidation. So, it is called a whispered pectoriloquy.

Another thing to consider is to do something called tactile fremitus. Take the hypothenar eminences and put them in the consolidation area. Normally, the vibration from the sound waves moving through the airway, pleura, and chest wall onto the hypothenar eminences depends on air. Also, whatever the fluid or substance that it is moving through. When sound waves move through a fluid consolidation, the vibrations intensify and will feel way more intensely in a patient with a consolidation than in a normal lung. So, they will have increased tactile fremitus.

So, these are some of the features of typical pneumonia.

Possible complications
When patients develop pneumonia, they can develop a couple of associated complications. Suppose they have

pneumonia in the left lower lobe, all locked up with the bacterium pus. That will cause localized inflammation so that the capillaries become leaky, invasive, and dilated, and fluid will start leaking into the pleural space. If the fluid leaks into the pleural space around that area of pneumonia, that is called a parapneumonic effusion. Sometimes, it can get locked up, and some bacteria spread contiguously into the space, making it a loculated appearance. So, there are two potential complications,

- a sterile inflammation around the pneumonia, or
- a lot of inflammation with a lot of loculated bacteria and pus within the pleural cavity.

The first one is called a parapneumonic effusion. Then, there is the other one, where there is a loculated type of pus infection within the pleural cavity, spreading from a localized area of pneumonia; this is called an empyema.

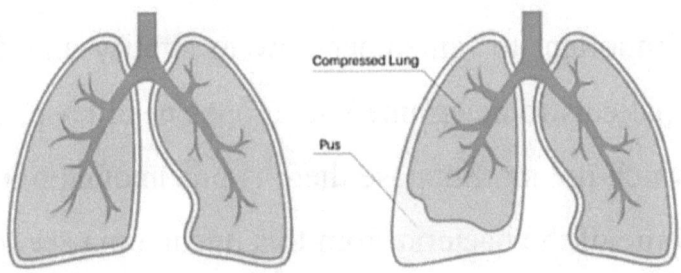

Sometimes, if the patient has many anaerobes, maybe Staphylococcus or Klebsiella - in those situations, they can have an infection in the lungs. However, the bacteria get smart, especially anaerobes, and those anaerobes start walling off the bacteria. Then they can get an infection where they have a big cavity filled with all this pus and bacteria. When they have this cavitation in the lungs, where there is the ability for the anaerobes or Klebsiella or Staphylococcus to wall themselves off, this is a lung abscess. It is another potential complication to remember with patients who have pneumonia.

The other thing is that as they start causing inflammation and infection of multiple alveoli and bronchial, they just continue to keep spreading; this is very common with bronchopneumonia, but as they start causing multiple alveoli, like diffuse alveolar damage to occur, they can lead to Acute Respiratory Distress Syndrome (ARDS).

It is important to remember how to stratify and diagnose these patients to determine which ones need hospitalization and which do not. Suppose there is pneumonia in a patient, and some of the bacteria from this pneumonia seed into the circulation. Furthermore, if they seed into the circulation, it causes bacteremia. Bacteremia does not necessarily mean sepsis, but if it seeds into the circulation and starts causing potential organ failure, then it might be getting into that kind of sepsis criteria, especially if the patient is having hypoxemia, low blood pressure, tachycardia, tachypnea, fevers. So, it is getting to that range of sepsis if a patient with pneumonia starts seeding into the actual circulatory system, causing And, when these pathogens get out, it potentially causes a low blood or low mean arterial pressure. In the patient, as we stop perfusing organs such as the kidneys, the liver, the brain, and multiple other organs, it can lead to multi-system organ failure.

Moreover, starts altering the normal coagulation system and decreasing the number of important platelets to form clots. Then, it starts consuming them to make a bunch of different clots, and there is the chance of bleeding, a situation called disseminated intravascular coagulation (DIC). So, it is important to remember that patients who develop pneumonia have a very high risk of sepsis, especially going down the road of septic shock.

Chapter Four: Diagnostics of Pneumonia.

So, a patient comes into the emergency department or clinic and presents with a cough, shortness of breath, fever, or is working hard to breathe, or they are complaining of that, and the rest of their heart rate is up. It is audible to hear of consolidation on their physical exam; they have a productive cough and pleuritic chest pain. Alternatively, maybe they just have atypical - low-grade fevers, respiratory tract infections like headaches, sore throat, nasal congestion, runny nose, and maybe a small quantity of myalgia or arthralgias.

Whenever a patient comes like that and thinks about the risk of pneumonia, such as the etiologies and pathophysiology, the next thing is to determine: Is this a community-acquired or a hospital-acquired? There are a couple of different things to remember for community-acquired pneumonia. It was acquired within the community, up to less than two days in the hospital. It is important because it determines the risk of what types of bugs, bacteria, and pathogens the patient will most likely use that degree of suspicion to say, 'It is likely CAP, and can use this particular antibiotic regimen.' However, if it is over two days in the hospital, it cannot be the same bug; it might be different. So, changing the antibiotic regimen is important.

When patients develop pneumonia within the community, it often tends to be a kind of lobar pneumonia. Moreover, there is a very specific pathogen in patients greater than 65 years of age and the aged, most common in nursing home facilities. It is the most common one, the Streptococcus pneumonia. A second line would be Haemophilus influenza, Moraxella catarrhalis, and COPD patients.

Conversely, HAP is when the patients have been in the hospital for over two days. Moreover, this could be in the hospital; they got a tube down their airway, intubated, for instance, VAP, the most common subset of HAP. This type of pneumonia is usually broncho, involving the bronchi, the bronchioles, and a part of the alveoli. Moreover, it is more scattered in that sense. Often, for these patients with HAP, the very specific types of pathogens to remember are generally MRSA and Pseudomonas. It is important to understand because, in the hospital, there are multi-drug-resistant pathogens.

When established, whether it is a HAP or a CAP based on the prior discussion, that can help determine the antibiotic regimen. In that instance, assessing the patient gives a certain degree of confidence that they have pneumonia. Next will be maybe getting some imaging. Thus, what are some of the labs that could be ordered for the patient? Alternatively, maybe presented with labs, the kind of clinical context, the clinical features, and based upon it being CAP or HAP, which types of labs are more suggestive or better?' Often, it is not that many; although there are many extra labs, maybe they are not super critical.

So, one of the things to consider is if they are presenting with features of upper respiratory tract infections. So, if they have any features of upper respiratory tract infections, get a respiratory viral panel because it will help look for influenza. Maybe it will help to rule out some type of SARS-CoV-2, like COVID-19 and RSV. The other thing is, frequently, just get some basic blood work for the patient. If they have this pneumonia, it will activate their immune system.

Moreover, if they activate their immune system, it will cause an immune response. It can release all those cytokines. It will activate their bone marrow and increase white blood cell production. So, expect an increase in their white blood cells, whether lymphocytes are more viral or neutrophils more bacterial, and order a complete blood count (CBC). That could be one potential thing. The other thing is that these infections can sometimes cause multi-system organ failure. If concerned about multi-system organ failure, then it could concern sepsis. So sometimes what can happen is to check maybe a basic metabolic panel (BMP). So, while checking their BMP, search for any evidence of an acute kidney injury, increasing their blood urea nitrogen (BUN), or any increase in the creatinine; this gives more about concern for organ failure. It could be potentially helpful that the BMP also shows low sodium. If a patient presents with low sodium who is aged, a smoker, immunocompromised, and has some type of exposure to contaminated water sources, then think about Legionella.

Sometimes, some of these pathogens can get into the bloodstream, and then they can get filtered across the kidney and into the urine. Specifically, some of their antigens can be tested. So we can test the urinary antigens. So, test the urinary antigens specifically for Strep-pneumo and Legionella. So these are some of the things to potentially start with a CBC to look for leukocytosis, a BMP to look for any acute kidney injury or hyponatremia (acute kidney injury be more concerning for early sepsis, hyponatremia suggestive of Legionella), and then consider the urinary antigens to look for Strep pneumonia or Legionella.

Sometimes, this inflammation can work on the liver, and when it works on the liver, it may cause the liver to increase C-reactive protein (CRP) production. Other times, some of these pathogens may get into the bloodstream and cause a kind of injury to the liver and cause a bump in the liver function tests (LFTs). Furthermore, one of the things to consider is that in a patient who has hyponatremia, nausea, vomiting, diarrhea, is an older person, is a smoker, or is immunocompromised, and some type of contaminated water source, it is Legionella. Thus, with hyponatremia and increased LFTs, consider Legionella.

If concerned that the patient is developing sepsis, get blood cultures. So consider also testing the blood to ensure the pathogen has not seeded into the circulatory system. Checking blood cultures may also be a good thing. Then, get the sputum cultures to determine the specific pathogen type. Sputum cultures may also be helpful to take and pull some of the sputum out. Suck some of that sputum out and then put it into a tube and then send that off to be tested for culture. So, with what is called a sputum culture, that will help narrow down the antibiotics.

With the labs, the major ones that would be worth considering are the CBC, blood cultures, sputum cultures, and respiratory viral panel. And then, potentially, a BMP will look for hyponatremia with increased LFTs and think about lesions.

Imaging

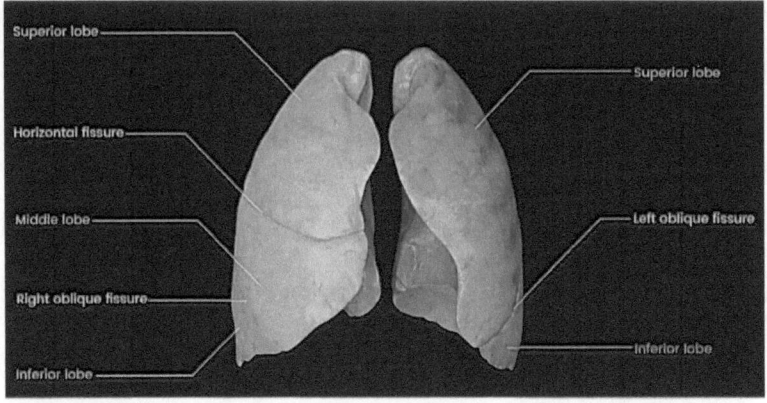

Imaging is potentially more superior and important. There are different things the actual image would suggest off the chest X-ray if present, such as if it is a lobar, interstitial, or bronchial. Also, there are other ways that we can define pneumonia, considering microbe acquisition and location. So, the actual type of pneumonia based upon location, we can define them as

- lobar,
- Bronchopneumonia and
- interstitial.

Lobar pneumonia occupies one of the lobes of the lung; it could be a right upper lobe, a right middle lobe, a right lower lobe, a left lower lobe, or left upper lower pneumonia, mostly due to streptococcus pneumonia. So, lobar pneumonia is situated in one of the lobes. If it is bronchial, it involves the bronchi and bronchioles scattered bilaterally, like patches.

The bronchopneumonia involves the bronchi, bronchioles, and some of the alveoli. So it will be very patchy, and it will be extended, kind of scattered throughout the lungs, with patchy opacities that are visible bilaterally. Moreover, the microbes responsible if it is hospital-acquired are usually

MRSA or Pseudomonas. However, if it is community-acquired, that is a different situation. It could be due to Staphylococcus aureus, streptococcus pneumonia, Haemophilus influenza, and Klebsiella for community-acquired bronchopneumonia.

The interstitial involves the interstitial spaces, and the pathogen is not infecting the lung parenchyma itself but causing infection in the interstitial spaces. Moreover, this is very common with atypical pneumonia caused by Mycoplasma, Chlamydia, Legionella and viruses. The most common is Mycoplasma, especially in young children, college dorms or dorm rooms, and in very close contact or occupied spaces.

For the imaging, what kind of imaging do we get? Do we get a chest X-ray or a Computed Tomography (CT) scan? A chest X-ray should often be the initial test whenever a patient comes in with symptoms like shortness of breath, pruritic chest pain, purling cough, or anything similar. The X-ray gives ease of access and will be quick to get done. The only time it is recommended to do a CT is if it is unclear what is going on off their chest X-ray if their chest X-ray is inconclusive while treating them for pneumonia, if they are not getting better, and if they are immunocompromised. So, the three reasons to get a CT include,

- chest X-ray is inconclusive, but there is a high degree of suspicion that it is pneumonia,
- while treating them for pneumonia, they are not getting better and
- they are immunocompromised, and there is suspicion that they may have some type of weird pneumonia that is worthy of taking a better look.

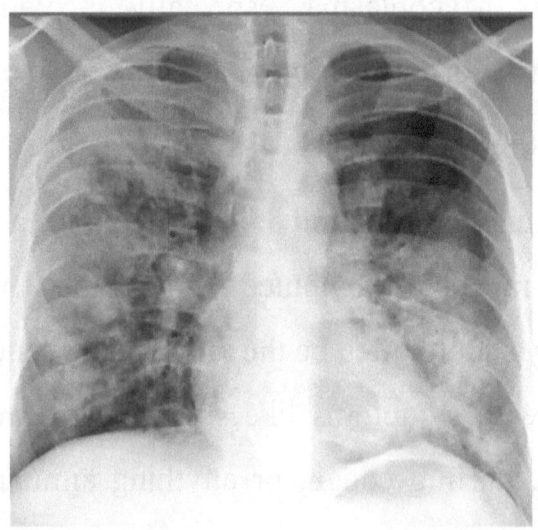

The image above is from a patient who has Broncho pneumonia. It is not situated in a particular lobe; some areas have patchy consolidation. So, it appears like a patchy bilateral consolidation in both lungs, common in outpatients with Staphylococcus, streptococcus, Hemophilus, and Klebsiella. If it is hospital-acquired, consider MRSA and Pseudomonas.

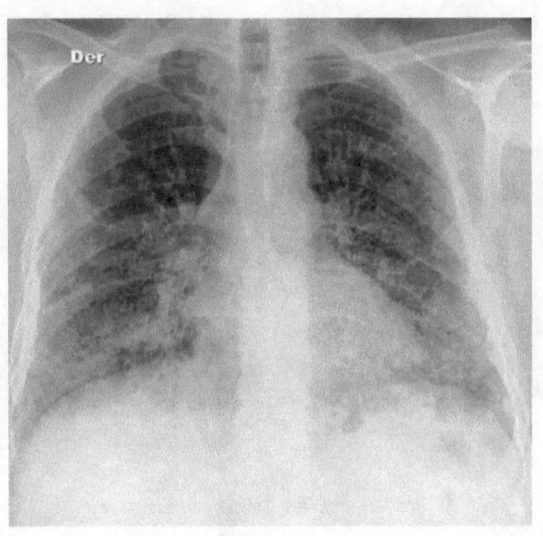

The image above is another conventional chest X-ray for a patient with headaches, nasal congestion, rhinorrhea, sore throat, ear aches with bullous meningitis. They had some low-grade fevers and arthralgias. They may be young and live in a dormitory, so consider Mycoplasma or chlamydia. Alternatively, if the reports said contaminated water sources in an aged young individual who smokes are immunosuppressed and others, then consider Legionella or viruses. However, the image shows a fine, threading-like appearance that almost resembles a ground glass type. It has that kind of ground glass opacities but fine reticular markings that move from the hilum outward towards the pleura. It is a classic example of interstitial pneumonia, which would be on differential for Mycoplasma, chlamydia, Legionella, and viruses.

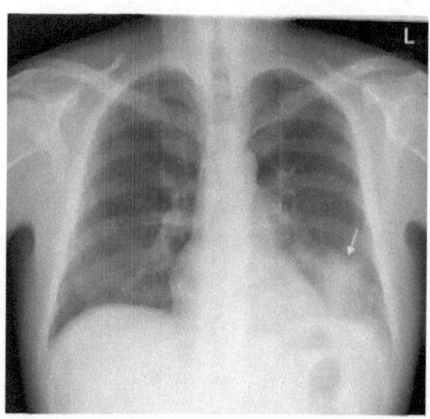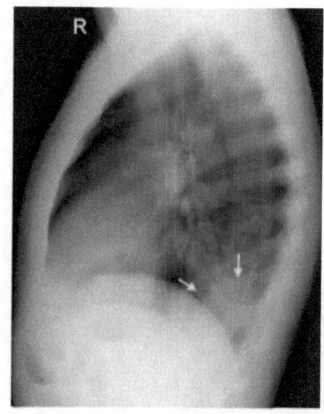

The images above describe a Posterior to Anterior (PA) and lateral chest X-ray. That deserves another question on which type of X-ray to put into the thing. In comparison, APs can sometimes distort the anatomy and do not provide the best clinical picture. PAs will be good pictures that will enhance the chest wall and show pathology, and lateral X-rays are good because sometimes they cannot show those lower lobes on a PA view. Thus, putting them in a lateral X-ray can give them that lower lobe view, which is nice. So, PA and lateral chest X-ray will be the best tests to do if there are options to pick between the chest X-rays. PA-lateral because PA gives information about the upper lobes and maybe a small amount of the right middle lobe, but the lower lobe sometimes can be hidden, and then it gets that better on the lateral chest X-ray. So, the image above shows the right upper lobes look good, the left upper lobe looks good, and the right middle lobe looks good, but cannot show the right lower lobe. However, on the left lower lobe it shows some opacity because it obscures the edge of the heart, like that left heart border, and might be missing some of the lower parts going down behind the diaphragm portion. So, the lateral image by the side shows a consolidated area on the left lower lobe. Thus, that shows the patient has left lower lobe pneumonia. So, that could be a strep pneumonia.

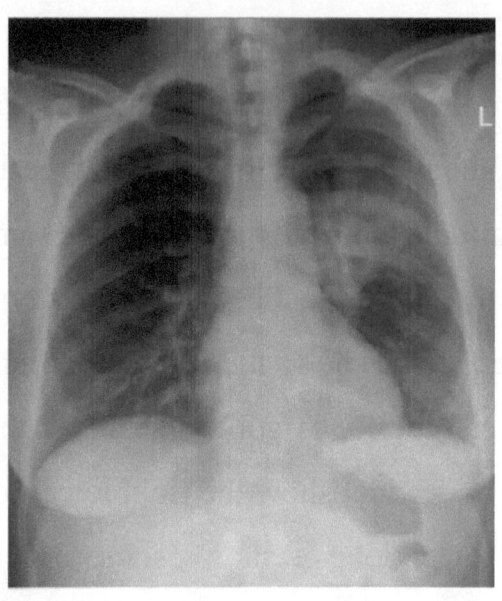

From the X-ray image above, the right upper lobe and right lower lobe look clean. It is easy to pick up the right heart border kind of left heart border and also make it out, and no opacity of the left lower lobe, but there is some sort of obscuring near the left portion of the mediastinum, near the aorta and the pulmonary knob. It obscures the left upper lobe, making it look hazy and pacified. That shows a left upper lobe pneumonia or a lobar pneumonia.

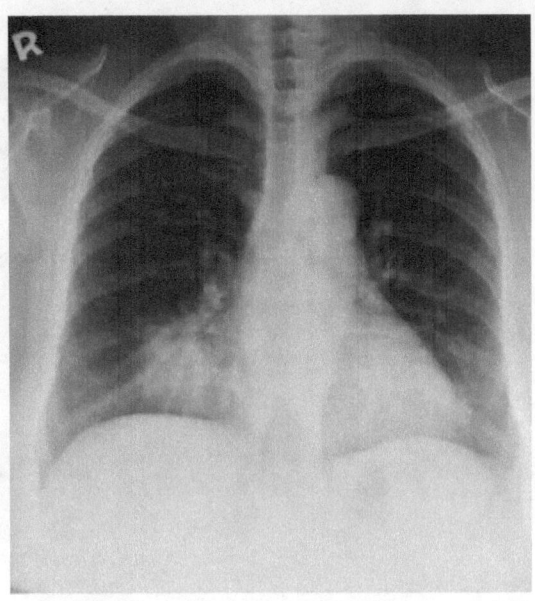

From the image, the right upper lobe and left upper lobe look clean, showing the left heart border and the left lower lobe looking relatively good. However, looking at that right border, it is not easy to make out completely, and there is a little opacity or hazy consolidation there on that right middle lobe portion. That is right, middle lobe pneumonia.

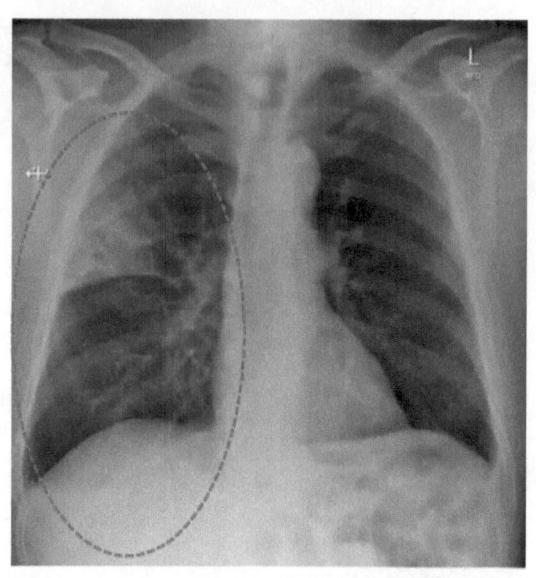

In the image above, the left upper and lower lobes are clean. It is easier to see the nice and right heart border. It shows the patient does not have right middle lobe pneumonia. However, a lateral view can give a better view of the right lower lobe and left lower lobe. However, something does pop out, like a sore thumb on the right upper lobe opacity. It does appear like a horizontal and oblique fissure, and there is a little fissure bulging there. Then, there is the opacity involving the right upper lobe.

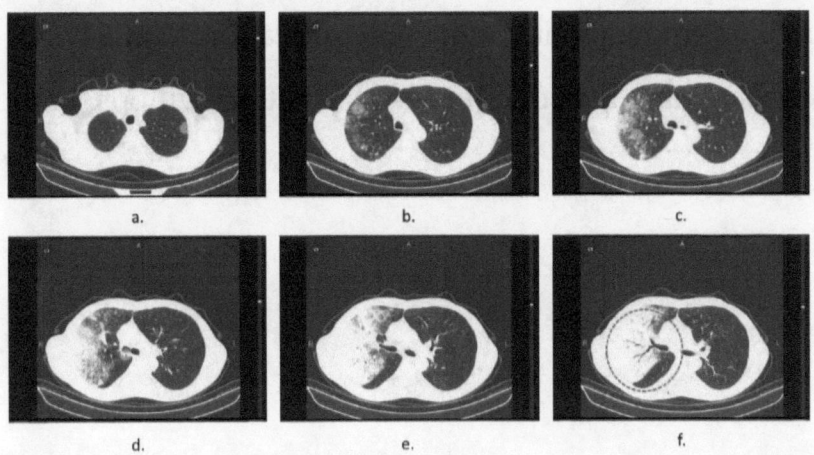

a.   b.   c.

d.   e.   f.

This next type of image is a CT. It is the best for pneumonia but is usually reserved for conditions where there is not enough information about the patient from the chest X-ray, such as if they are not getting better with antibiotics or immunocompromised. Looking at the CT image of the right lung (b), it is easy to observe a kind of hazy opacities in the right hemithorax. In comparison to the left, it looks nice and aerated. Moving further (c to f), it is getting worse with more opacities. The image (f) shows some interesting results. The bronchus coming off and moving into this consolidation showed it is open, demonstrating there is much air moving into it, and then it stops like a cutoff here. These are called air bronchograms, which are very characteristic of pneumonia. The consolidation and opened-up air-filled cavities moving into the consolidation, called an air bronchogram, are consistent with a patient with pneumonia.

Chapter Five: Treatment of Pneumonia

We will discuss this, particularly focusing on the antibiotics used to treat the infection because it is an infection of the actual lung tissue, so the primary focus should be treating it. There are a lot of supportive measures that come into it as well, obviously treating potentially the hypoxemia the patient may have and the work of breathing. The focus is on the antibiotics, but the antibiotics depend on the type of pneumonia the patient has. Moreover, that depends on stratifying these patients and determining their need for outpatient care, in-hospital care but not in the ICU, and then ICU-level care. Alternatively, they have been in the hospital for a couple of days, more than two days, more than 48 hours, and they have developed pneumonia, so they have a HAP. So, when a patient comes in, it is essential to determine if it is a community-acquired pneumonia that can go home to the floor or the ICU. The way to do that is something called the CURB-65 score.

- Confusion: Remember that if a patient gets pneumonia, one of the complications is that the bacteria can seed into the bloodstream, causing a decrease in their main opportunity or perfusion. They do not perfuse the brain

51

as well; they do not perfuse the kidney; they do not perfuse the liver. They develop multi-system organ failure. One of the first things for aged individuals is that they develop confusion or altered mental status, and this is due to the septic feature. So, if they are already presenting with sepsis, that is a concerning sign. So, confusion is a very concerning sign.

– Uremia: this is the increase in the urea, particularly their BMP, and whenever we say the uremia is present, it is mainly estimated to be greater than 20. In this situation, that would be concerning. That would tell that there was an acute kidney injury, decreasing the perfusion to their kidneys potentially. So, they have an acute kidney injury, and that is a concerning sign, meaning that they need to be hospitalized.

– Respiration: if their respiratory rate is high, like greater than 30 breaths per minute, they are breathing super fast and tachycardic.

– Blood pressure: With the mean arterial pressure dropping, or they are hypotensive, that is a problem. So, if their blood pressure is low, especially about two particular parameters: If their systolic blood pressure is less than 90 millimeters of mercury or if their diastolic blood pressure is less than 60 millimeters, this is a concerning sign.

– Patients who are greater than 65 years of age are obviously at higher risk of worse outcomes. Thus, it is worth assuming that as people get older, the immune system is becoming compromised. People have impaired mucous ciliary clearance and are likely to have other comorbidities that put them at higher risk. So, if the patients are 65 or older, they are at high risk.

Furthermore, summing up all the points, if the patients have one of these, they get a point. Moreover, risk-stratifying based on their score,

- Their score is between zero and one, (0-1) a patient with a relatively confident level, does not have sepsis, multi-system organ failure, and can decompensate. So, it is okay to send these patients home; that would be a CAP outpatient.

- If their score is two, being slightly more concerned for this patient is okay. It is a patient that could potentially decompensate, and they need more observation;

maybe not an ICU level of care, but they need some observation. So, this is a CAP, but this will be a non-ICU admission.

- A patient must have some concern if they have three plus (3 plus). They have a very high mortality rate and should not be sent home. The patients may not be sent to a non-ICU; they need very close observation and very aggressive care. These are patients who have community-acquired pneumonia and require ICU-level care.

After the patients are risk-stratified, determining those with high mortality, low mortality, and intermediate mortality provides a sequence to treat these patients accordingly to CAP outpatient, CAP non-ICU, CAP ICU, and then HAP.

CAP outpatients

With CAP outpatients, remember that in these particular populations, it deals mainly with atypical, possibly even Strep pneumonia. So, what covers the Strep pneumonia also covers the atypicals pretty well.

The first option to consider in these patients would be macrolides (e.g., azithromycin) or doxycycline (doxy), one of those actual tetracyclines we can also consider. The second option would be respiratory fluoroquinolone but do not do this first because of high resistance. This option is only recommended if a patient has an underlying comorbidity that puts them at high risk or they have gotten antibiotics in less than 90 days. If they have, then maybe they may have higher resistance. Thus, a respiratory fluoroquinolone may work well if they have had antibiotics in the last 90 days or if comorbidity is present.

If a patient has community-acquired pneumonia and is in the hospital but in observation and not in an ICU setting, try to do a respiratory fluoroquinolone; that would be an option as monotherapy. The other option is to consider doing a macrolide or doxy plus a beta-lactam. Moreover, the preferred beta-lactam depends on the hospital ward, but the most preferred agent is often Ceftriaxone. For a patient in the ICU with community-acquired pneumonia, in that situation, do somewhat of the same steps above but then get rid of the doxycycline. Thus, the two options:

(1) One is to do a macrolide (azithromycin), or
(2) Do a respiratory fluoroquinolone.

The only difference is adding a beta-lactam to one of these particular regimens. Preferred Ceftriaxone does not mean a lack of choice; sometimes, use Augmentin, which is amoxicillin clavulanate, as another option, or ampicillin-sulbactam, also known as Unasyn.

- HAP is generally greater than two days in the hospital. So whether this is with a tube down the airway or not, once in the hospital for two days or more, and the patient has pneumonia, it is now a HAP. It covers different bugs; the first is MRSA, generally treated with Vancomycin, and another option is Linezolid. For Pseudomonas aeruginosa. use the piperacillin-tazobactam, (sometimes Pip-tazo or Zosyn). The other option is cefepime. The other option to consider is aminoglycosides (Tobramycin, Gentamicin, Amy casein), but try to avoid these because they are harsh on the kidneys. Another possible option is Aminoglycosides, but try to avoid these as an option. The other thing that to also consider is if a patient is HIV positive and their CD4 count is less than 200 and may have PJP, there are some options to treat. One such option to treat them with is Bactrim

(trimethoprim-sulfamethoxazole). The only other thing to possibly add on is a respiratory fluoroquinolone like levofloxacin or moxifloxacin suspected that the patient has Legionella.

– Another is aspiration. Compared to real-life aspiration pneumonia, the kind of pathogens are usually anaerobes because of the lung. However, the lung is usually aerated, very aerobic, and filled with oxygen, so it will be hard for an anaerobe to survive in the lungs. Therefore, unless the patient has a lung abscess or an empyema, do not treat for anaerobic infections with these particular bugs.

Clindamycin would be one potential option for this treatment, and another may be Augmentin(amoxicillin-clavulanate). Another option to consider is metronidazole plus a beta-lactam. However, because the lung is so aerated, do not treat aspiration pneumonia with these pathogens. Treat it as though it is a HAP or a CAP, same treatment unless they have a lung abscess or an empyema, then treat with clindamycin, Augmentin, beta-lactam, and metronidazole.

Remember, the potential treatment of pneumonia is prevention. It is with the pneumococcal vaccination (PCV). So PCV 13 is generally at 2, 4, 6, and 12 to 15 months of age. Then, the Pneumococcal Polysaccharide Vaccine (PPSV 23) vaccinations are given at 65 or older or if they have a lot of underlying conditions that put them at risk in patients 2 to 64 years of age.

Chapter Six: Case Study

Suppose we have a 72-year-old female presented to the clinic with a purulent cough, dyspnea, rigors, and progressive confusion. Past medical history is significant for COPD, diabetes, and HIV. So we know this patient is going to have pneumonia, but some of the features that are suggestive of pneumonia and are concerning is

- she has a purulent cough and has a purulent sputum production,
- she has dyspnea, which could be indicative of much consolidation, causing hypoxemia to some degree,
- she has rigors, which could be due to the fevers from a bacterial type of source here, and
- she has progressive confusion, maybe kind of suggesting to some degree that she has some type of organ dysfunction. She may not be allowing for proper perfusion of the brain. Especially in aged individuals, we can see that, so concerning finding there.

Her past medical issues are also kind of supportive of worse lung problems; COPD can cause a lot of nasty bugs. Also, diabetes makes her more immunocompromised, plus she is

HIV positive, and that also makes her super immunocompromised. Being immunocompromised, maybe due to HIV, means the patient may not be able to have the immune system response that she needs to fight off any kind of normal pathogens in her airway. So, these are very concerning findings.

So, she has many risk factors that increase the risk of her having some type of pneumonia or COPD. Again, a lot of thickening secretions, many bronchospasms, and again, because of the inability to beat the mucociliary apparatus, that is a problem.

Physical examination
She is 72, which makes her a little bit more aged and again reduces the amount of cilia, reduces that up kind of like process there.

Physical examination:

Vitals	BP	80/50		
	HR	110		
	RR	32		
	Temp	38.3°C (101°F)		
	SpO2	84%	FiO2	60%

Her vitals are not very good at all; her BP is 80 over 50, so she is hypotensive. She is slightly tachycardic, so her heart rate is 110, and her respiratory rate is 32. Her temperature is elevated, so she has a temperature of 101 degrees Fahrenheit. She is febrile, tachycardic, and mildly hypotensive. On top of that, her SpO2 is bad, so she is on 84 percent, and she is already on FiO2 of 60, so she must be on some type of supplemental oxygen source giving her 60% FiO2. Maybe some type of high-flow nasal cannula.

So, in general, this is a concerning finding for this patient. She is hypoxemic on oxygen supplementation, febrile, tachycardic, and hypotensive.

When we examine the patient's chest, we want to think about signs of consolidation. So, things will alter the process of auscultating, tactile fremitus, auscultating the process of these sounds or whispers, and percussion.

So, to find concerning findings of consolidation, we listen for bronchial breath sounds, which means there is consolidation as the bronchus is trying to run into the smaller bronchial. It is running into a consolidative area, so it is possible to hear the breath sounds proximal to that consolidation, such as bronchial breath sounds. When percussing, generally, anything that is more fluid-filled or pus-filled in this kind of case will give a more dull type of percussion, and it will be louder on tactile fremitus. So, they will have an increased tactile fremitus. They will also have positive bronchophony, egophony, and whisper pectoriloquy on their specialized tests.

Chest **What are Signs of Consolidation?**
Bronchial breath sounds
Dullness to percussion
Increased tactile fremitus
Bronchophony
Egophony
Whispered Pectoriloquy

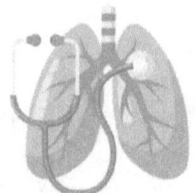

These are all findings that are supportive of consolidation for this patient.

Diagnosis

The next phase involves the diagnosis, which could be pneumonia. We can get a bunch of different labs and imaging, and starting with a CBC would not be a bad idea in the comprehensive metabolic panel (CMP).

Diagnosis

CBC   Leukocytosis

CMP   BUN   ~30
         LFTs   Normal
         [Na]   Normal

Blood Cultures   H.Flu, Strep PNA
Sputum Cultures   PJP, H.Flu, Strep PNA

CD4   <200

Images   B/L patchy consolidations

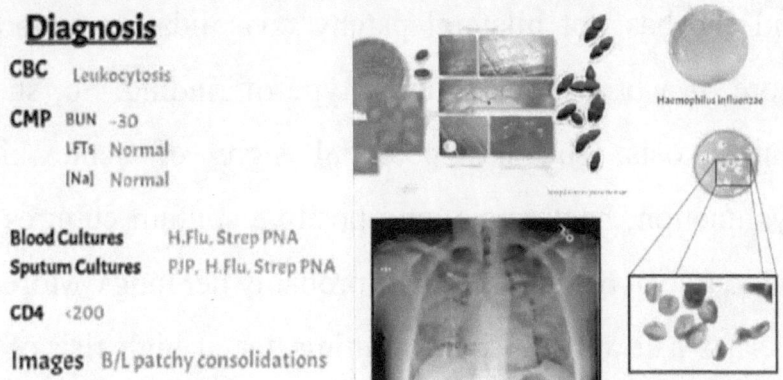

Haemophilus influenzae

Pneumocystis Jiroveci Pneumonia

The results of the CBC showed that the patient has leukocytosis, so she has an elevated white count, which may be supportive of an infectious etiology. CMP shows a bun of 30, showing she has an elevated bun, and her creatinine was also slightly elevated. Her LFTs and sodium are normal, which is important for Legionella.

Her blood cultures came back positive for Haemophilus influenza and Streptococcus pneumonia. Then, her sputum cultures were positive for PJP, H. flu, and Streptococcus pneumonia. Her CD4 count, because she is HIV positive, is less than 200, and her imaging on chest X-rays showed bilateral patchy consolidations.

So, she has a bacterial infection, both bacteremic and mnemonic. She has HIV with a very, very low CD4 count,

63

and she has got bilateral patchy consolidation supporting more of a bronchopneumonia type of finding. So, she has leukocytosis; she has potential signs of acute kidney dysfunction, bacteremia, and positive sputum cultures, and the source of her bacteremia is probably her lungs. Moreover, she has a low CD4 count, putting her at high risk of PJP, which she is positive for, and her lungs are supportive of consolidated findings. So, she has bad pneumonia secondary to Strep pneumo and H flu. And then she has also got a small amount of PJP due to her CD4 HIV being less than 200.

Recall that there are three types of radiographic pneumonia,

1. bronchopneumonia,
2. lobar,
3. interstitial pneumonia.

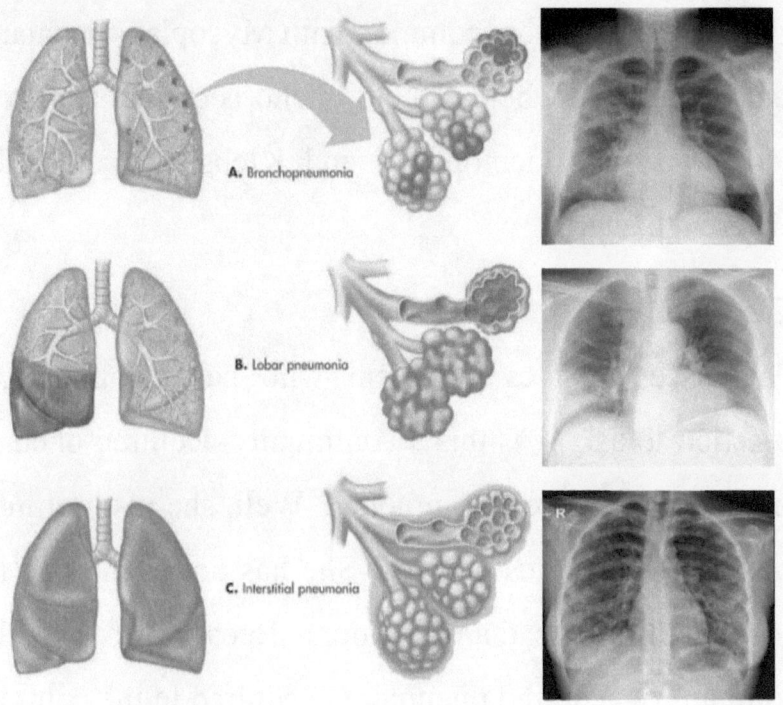

A. Bronchopneumonia

B. Lobar pneumonia

C. Interstitial pneumonia

Lobar bronchopneumonia is usually like socked-in pneumonia; it is consolidated, potentially usually one lobe or two lobes. Generally, it would be like a right middle or lower lobe kind of pneumonia, usually socked up. The common type is the pneumococcal pneumonia.

Broncho pneumonia is more scattered, bilateral, and patchy and usually involves the smaller bronchioles and alveolar tissue; many different bugs can cause that.

And then the last is interstitial pneumonia. It appears a lot like interstitial infiltrates and usually like reticular nodular kind of opacification, common with Mycoplasma, chlamydia, and Legionella, whereas the broncho is common with staph and strap and Haemophilus and Klebsiella, and a lot of different bacteria.

Treatment

This case involves a patient who has pneumonia. The question to ask is, is this a community-acquired pneumonia or hospital-acquired pneumonia? Well, she just got into the hospital and has just arrived. She has not even been in the hospital for more than 48 hours. Because of that, this is community-acquired pneumonia acquired in the community since she has not even been in the hospital for very long at all.

The next consideration is what level of care the patient may require and how to determine the level of care. Remember the CURB-65 score. So, what out of these does she have, and then based upon that, what puts her at high risk?

CURB-65 score	C	Confusion
	U	Uremia> 20
	R	RR>30
	B	BP <90/60
	65	>65 years

From her CURB-65 score, She has confusion seen in her HPI. She does have uremia; her urea was greater than 20(30). Her respiratory rate was about 34, so she has tachypnea, which supports that. Her BP's are soft, so she had an 80 over 50. She is 72 and over 65 years of age. She has all of those findings, so generally, when someone has potentially high findings, like three or more, that is very concerning and requires ICU-level care. So, this patient needs to go to the ICU.

In the ICU, start her on antibiotics because, obviously, the core, the source of this, is bacterial pneumonia. There are so many different types of bacteria that can cause pneumonia, but likely hers is, again, because she is 72, and the most common cause of community-acquired pneumonia in aged individuals is Streptococcus pneumonia. Moreover, on top of that, she has COPD and diabetes, which puts her at high risk for Haemophilus influenza, and she has HIV, which puts her at risk of PJP. She has a multi-bacterial type of polymicrobial pneumonia and evidence of sepsis, too. So, she is also septic.

To treat this patient, albeit excluding sepsis at this point and only treating pneumonia, the kind of antibiotics to put her on is based upon her CURB-65 score and putting her in ICU level care. That would include a beta-lactam and a macrolide, generally going to be the first thing to do, or we can do a fluoroquinolone and a beta-lactam of some type. These would generally be what to start on treatment for the patient. So get them started on this, and then when their cultures come back, narrow down according to what is best. Nevertheless, a beta-lactam, a macrolide, and a fluoroquinolone would put her in this kind of ICU-level category.

If she is becoming septic, potentially change the antibiotics up slightly. Often, patients just get put on something like Vancomycin and piperacillin-tazobactam. However, the best thing is that she would be appropriate with a beta-lactam antibiotic such as Ceftriaxone and a macrolide such as azithromycin.

In this particular situation, if that was not appropriate, use a beta-lactam like Ceftriaxone and a fluoroquinolone if there were concerns that she had MRSA. The cultures came back with no MRSA, so treat her with Vancomycin if her cultures came back positive for Pseudomonas aeruginosa, or if concerned about that, then put her on something like pip-tazo. She does not have that; treat her for what we would suspect based upon the guidelines discussed earlier and what her sputum cultures and blood cultures came back positive for a beta-lactam and a macrolide or a beta-lactam and a fluoroquinolone would be appropriate here.

There is one other thing that she did test positive for, which is PJP, and PJP generally, we should treat these patients with Bactrim in this particular situation, which is trimethoprim-sulfamethoxazole.

The next consideration is that when it is pneumonia, one of the complications of pneumonia is things like ARDS and possibly peritonic effusions that can lead to empyemas. There are a lot of different things that can happen with this potential disease. One of the worst-case scenarios is that the patient can seed some of the bacteria into their systemic circulation, which can cause worsening features of hypotension, tachycardia, severe fevers, and sometimes become refractory to fluids and vasopressors. We can see the patient becoming septic and going into septic shock. From the report, the patient does have features of sepsis and some degree of septic shock because they lower the blood pressure and have the potential for organ dysfunction. So, this patient is at the point of septic shock, which is concerning.

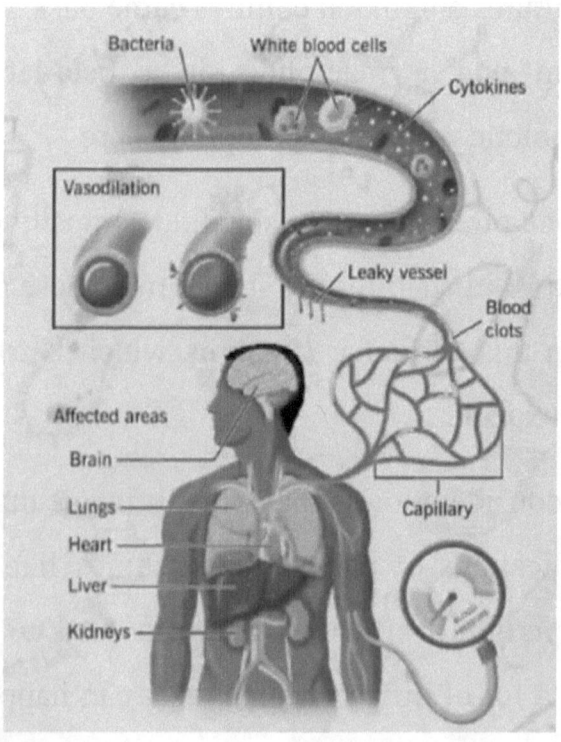

Again, treat the patient accordingly for septic shock, such as putting them on vasopressors and fluids, with a minimal kind of fluid approach. And then, on top of that, considering things such as antibiotics for their pneumonia. So, treating them for pneumonia, vasopressors to support their blood pressure, plus or minus a small quantity of fluids, just being careful not to overload them with fluids.

Matching

- Using the term "strep pneumonia", which would be more of a support of strep pneumonia, it is the most common cause of community-acquired pneumonia in aged individuals, and that is Streptococcus pneumonia.
- For Staph aureus, think about post-influenza and IV drug abuse. MRSA is related to a hospital-acquired pneumonia type of pathogen that's very dangerous.
- Next are H. flu and Moraxella; consider COPD and some bronchiectasis.
- For Klebsiella, consider alcoholics' CNS disease and depression. Anything that increases the risk of aspiration would be Klebsiella.
- For Pseudomonas, think that immunocompromised or immunosuppressed in cystic fibrosis is also a harbinger for Pseudomonas.

- Mycoplasma is considered young, healthy, and close-quarter living, especially in dormitories.
- For Legionella, consider contaminated water sources; they are a smoker, aged, and immunocompromised.
- For PJP, consider HIV/AIDS, CD4 count less than 200.
- Coccidioidomycosis is a fungus in the southwestern United States, including California.
- Histoplasmosis occurs in bird or bat droppings, infecting patients during the spelunking events in the Ohio and Mississippi River Valley.
- For Blastomycosis, consider the yeast from the Eastern United States.
- For anaerobic bacteria, consider situations of aspiration events.